FOOD & NUTRITION

The Basics of Raw Food

By

Jon T. Lange

Table of Contents
Chapter one

Chapter 2

Chapter 3

Chapter 4

Chapter 5

Introduction

In order to sustain general health and wellbeing, food and nutrition are essential components of human life. The food decisions we make directly affect our physical health, cognitive function, energy levels, and even emotional wellbeing. For healthy development, growth, and systemic health, proper nutrition is essential.

Food and nutrition are significant because they give the body the vital nutrients and energy it needs to perform at its best. Nutritional components, including carbohydrates, proteins, lipids, vitamins, and minerals, are essential for a number of physiological activities, including immunological response, metabolic processes, and tissue repair. A well-balanced diet offers an adequate and suitable supply of these nutrients. Each nutrient has a specific function in the body.

In addition to giving us the nutrition we require, food also promotes culture, social connection, and enjoyment. The act of cooking and eating together can encourage relationships and a sense of community. Traditional foods frequently enhance a sense of community and legacy. Food is an essential component of cultural identity.

A balanced and nourishing diet requires an understanding of the fundamental food groups. Fruits, vegetables, grains, meals high in protein, and dairy (or dairy substitutes) are generally considered to be the major food groups. Every category offers a special combination of nutrients required for good health. It is possible to consume a wide range of necessary nutrients by incorporating a variety of meals from each group.

Additionally, the importance of healthy eating for illness prevention cannot be overemphasized. Chronic conditions like heart disease, diabetes, and some forms of cancer have been related to a lower risk of a well-balanced diet. Adopting healthy eating habits and making informed food choices can help you stay healthy and lower your risk of developing these disorders.

Furthermore, the relationship between nutrition, mental health, and cognition is strong. The health of the brain and the control of mood are significantly influenced by specific nutrients such as omega-3 fatty acids, B vitamins, and antioxidants. An adequate diet promotes memory, cognition, and general mental health.

In general, eating and nutrition are crucial to human health and wellbeing. They contribute to the prevention of disease, boost cognitive function, improve quality of life, and offer the minerals and energy required for biological processes. Our physical and emotional health can benefit significantly from making thoughtful food decisions and adopting a balanced, nutrient-rich diet.

Chapter 1

What Are Food and Nutrition?

Food: Any substance taken by living things is referred to as food. This is normally done for hydration, energy, growth, and the maintenance of bodily processes. It contains both plant-based and animal-based foods that contain vital elements such as carbohydrates, proteins, lipids, vitamins, minerals, and water.

Nutrition: Nutrition is the process through which the body uses and acquires sustenance from food. It encompasses the ingesting, absorbing, assimilation, metabolism, and utilization of nutrients to support growth, development, health maintenance, and general well-being.

Nutrition involves the study of nutrients, their origins, functions, interactions, and the impact of dietary habits on human health. It involves comprehending how various foods and nutrients affect the physiological processes of the body and many elements of health, including physical, cognitive, and emotional well-being.

The area of nutrition is additionally concentrated on addressing specific dietary needs and concerns, such as vitamin shortages, chronic diseases, weight management, and supporting optimal health across several life phases, including infancy, childhood, adolescence, maturity, and older adults.

In conclusion, eating and consuming food for nourishment, health, growth, and total wellbeing are related ideas. Maintaining good health and avoiding problems linked to diet depend heavily on proper nutrition.

Benefits of Nutrition and Food

It is impossible to exaggerate the significance of food and nutrition because they are essential for preserving general health and wellbeing. Following are some of the main justifications for why nutrition and diet are crucial:

1. **Energy and Vitality:** Food gives the body the energy it needs to carry out daily activities, ensuring optimal energy levels and vitality. Fruits, vegetables, whole grains, and lean proteins are examples of nutrient-rich diets that provide the calories and nutrients needed to maintain biological functioning.

2. **Nutrient Supply**: Good nutrition assures the consumption of vital nutrients such as carbs, proteins, fats, vitamins, and minerals. These nutrients are necessary for development, growth, and the preservation of essential body processes. They boost the immune system, control metabolism, encourage good digestion, and facilitate a number of physiological activities.

3. **Disease Prevention**: A healthy, balanced diet is essential for preventing chronic conditions including diabetes, heart disease, and some forms of cancer. By supplying necessary antioxidants, fiber, and other advantageous chemicals, a diet rich in a range of fruits, vegetables, whole grains, and lean meats helps lower the chance of acquiring these illnesses.

4. **Weight Management**: An efficient diet is essential for preserving a healthy weight. A balanced diet, portion control, and regular exercise all aid in obtaining and maintaining a healthy body weight. It encourages a healthy balance between caloric intake and expenditure, avoiding weight gain and lowering the risk of obesity-related consequences.

5. **Cognitive Function**: Nutrition has an impact on both brain health and cognitive function. The correct growth and operation

of the brain depend on a number of nutrients, including vitamins, antioxidants, and omega-3 fatty acids. A nutritious diet can improve focus, concentration, memory, and general mental health.

6. Gut health and digestion are both impacted by good nutrition. A diet high in fiber helps with digestion, avoids constipation, and encourages a diverse and balanced gut microbiota. Numerous elements of health, such as immunity, mental health, and even weight control, have been related to the gut microbiome.

7. **Emotional Well-Being**: There is mounting proof that links diet and mental health. A nutritious diet that includes foods high in vitamins, minerals, and omega-3 fatty acids may help lower the risk of depression and anxiety as well as enhance mood.

8. Longevity and Quality of Life: A balanced diet and proper nutrition are linked to both a longer life expectancy and a higher quality of life. Proper nutrition promotes appropriate aging and a higher quality of life in later years by giving the body the nutrients it needs, lowering the risk of chronic diseases, and maintaining overall health.

In conclusion, nutrition and food have a critical role in sustaining the body's processes, preventing disease, preserving a healthy weight, enhancing cognitive function, and fostering general wellbeing. People may harness the advantages of appropriate nutrition and live a healthier and more meaningful life by making informed food decisions and forming healthy eating habits.

Main Food Groups

The following categories generally apply to the basic food groups in nutrition and food:

1. Fruits are the first food category and include a wide range of fruits, such as apples, bananas, strawberries, oranges, and more. Fruits are a natural source of low-fat, important nutrients and are high in vitamins, minerals, fiber, and antioxidants.

2. **Vegetables**: Some examples of vegetables are root vegetables like carrots and potatoes, leafy greens like spinach and kale, and cruciferous veggies like broccoli and cauliflower. They are an excellent source of fiber, phytochemicals, vitamins, and minerals. Consuming a diversity of vegetables can help guarantee that you are getting a wide array of nutrients.

3. **Grains**: Both whole and refined grains are included in the grain food group. All

portions of the grain, including the bran, germ, and endosperm, are present in whole grains like brown rice, quinoa, oats, and whole wheat bread, giving fiber, B vitamins, and minerals. The bran and germ of refined grains, such as white rice and white bread, have been removed, lowering their nutritional value.

4. **Protein-rich foods**: Both plant- and animal-based sources of protein fall under this category. Dairy products, meat, poultry, fish, and eggs are examples of animal-based foods. Legumes (beans, lentils), tofu, tempeh, and seitan, as well as some grains and seeds, are examples of plant-based foods. Protein helps people feel fuller longer and is necessary for the growth, maintenance, and repair of body tissues.

5. **Dairy:** This category includes dairy products such as milk, cheese, yogurt, and

more. Dairy products are a good source of protein, calcium, and vitamin D. Almond milk, soy milk, and coconut milk are plant-based alternatives for people who cannot consume dairy owing to lactose sensitivity or dietary preferences. These milks have been fortified with calcium and micronutrients.

It's crucial to remember that this classification may change depending on the cultural traditions or dietary restrictions used. Although they are not regarded as food groups, fats and oils are still a part of the diet. However, they should only be used in moderation, with an emphasis on better-for-you choices like olive oil, avocados, and almonds.

Eating a varied selection of foods from each of these food groups on a regular basis will ensure that you are consuming the essential nutrients needed for optimum health and well-being.

Vital Foodstuffs

The body cannot generate certain nutrients in sufficient amounts or sometimes at all, making them essential. To promote normal growth, development, and general health, these nutrients must be provided through diet or supplements. Following are some necessary nutrients along with their main purposes:

1. **Carbohydrates:** The body uses carbohydrates as its main energy source. They fuel the body's different processes as well as the brain, muscles, and other organs. Fruits, vegetables, whole grains, and legumes are excellent sources of carbs.

2. **Proteins**: Proteins play a crucial role in the development, maintenance, and repair of body tissues and cells. They are made up of amino acids, which are essential to many

biological activities. Meat, poultry, fish, eggs, dairy products, legumes, nuts, and seeds are examples of foods high in protein.

3. **Fats**: Dietary fats are necessary for maintaining good skin and hair, supplying energy, assisting in the absorption of fat-soluble vitamins, and protecting organs. Healthy unsaturated fats are preferred over saturated and trans fats and include those in avocados, nuts, seeds, and olive oil.

4. **Vitamins**: Vitamins are organic substances required for a number of body processes as well as good health. They are essential for the creation of energy, immune system performance, cell division, and the preservation of strong bones, skin, and eyes. The roles of individual vitamins vary, and they can be found in a variety of foods. Citrus fruits, for instance, are rich in vitamin C, while carrots and sweet potatoes are rich in vitamin A.

5. **Minerals:** Minerals are inorganic materials that are essential to preserving healthy biological functions. They participate in functions like fluid balance, nerve conduction, and bone development. Minerals like calcium, iron, zinc, magnesium, and potassium are examples of important minerals. Foods including dairy, leafy green vegetables, meat, beans, and whole grains provide these nutrients.

6. **Water:** Though frequently disregarded, water is necessary for life. Nearly every biological process, including digestion, nutrition absorption, waste elimination, temperature regulation, and joint lubrication, depends on it. For optimal health, it's important to stay hydrated, and water should always be your first choice.

Although fiber is not considered a nutrient, it is nevertheless an important part of a balanced diet and should not be overlooked. These are the main basic elements. Dietary fiber encourages regular bowel movements, aids in appropriate digestion, and increases feelings of fullness.

To ensure an appropriate intake of these vital nutrients, a well-balanced diet that consists of a variety of foods from several food categories is necessary. Individualized advice on dietary needs and nutritional requirements can be obtained by speaking with a medical expert or certified dietitian.

Chapter 2

Vegan and vegetarian diets

Two different dietary approaches that forgo using some animal products are vegetarian and vegan diets. Following is a summary of the culinary and nutritional benefits of vegetarian and vegan diets:

1. **Vegetarian Diet**: Vegetarians generally avoid eating seafood, meat, and fowl. Nevertheless, it may contain additional animal-derived goods, such as dairy, eggs, and honey, based on the tastes of the individual. Vegetarian diets can take many different forms:

Lacto-vegetarian: Includes dairy items but excludes meat, poultry, shellfish, and eggs.

Ovo-vegetarian: Includes eggs but excludes dairy, meat, poultry, and seafood.

Lacto-ovo-vegetarian: Includes dairy products and eggs but excludes meat, poultry, and seafood.

Pescatarian: Includes seafood and occasionally eggs but avoids meat, poultry, and dairy.

It can supply all the essential nutrients, including protein, carbs, lipids, vitamins, and minerals, for individuals who follow a well-planned vegetarian diet. Legumes, tofu, tempeh, seitan, and some grains and seeds are examples of plant-based sources of protein that can satisfy protein requirements. Fruits, vegetables, entire grains, nuts, and seeds all contain essential elements.

2. **Vegan Diet**: A vegan diet goes beyond vegetarianism by excluding the use of any animal products, including dairy, eggs, honey, meat, poultry, and fish. Vegans get all of their nutrients from plant-based foods alone. A well-balanced vegan diet can include all the necessary nutrients with

careful planning. Important factors include the following:

Protein: To meet protein needs, consume plant-based protein sources such as beans, tofu, tempeh, seitan, quinoa, and certain grains and seeds.

Vitamin B12: Vegans must guarantee appropriate consumption through fortified foods or supplements because this vitamin is largely found in animal sources.

Calcium: Leafy green vegetables, fortified plant-based milks, tofu, and some nuts and seeds are plant-based sources of calcium. Iron: Leafy green vegetables, legumes, fortified cereals, and dried fruits are plant-based sources of iron. Foods high in vitamin C improve iron absorption.

Omega-3 Fatty Acids: Flaxseeds, chia seeds, hemp seeds, and walnuts are plant-based sources of these crucial fatty acids for vegans. Alternately, there are supplements made of algae.

Vitamin D: Vegans have few food sources of this vitamin; therefore, it's critical to get enough sun exposure and consume fortified foods and pills.

Vegetarians and vegans must carefully monitor their nutrient consumption, particularly their intake of the vitamins B12, D, and omega-3 fatty acids. A certified dietitian or other healthcare provider can offer specialized advice on fulfilling nutritional requirements and avoiding deficits in these diets.

Additionally, as vegetarian and vegan diets often involve higher consumption of fiber, antioxidants, and plant-based components, they may provide additional health advantages such as a decreased risk of heart disease, some malignancies, and type 2 diabetes. To keep your health at its best while following these dietary patterns, you must make sure that your diet is well-planned and varied.

Diet free of gluten

A gluten-free diet forgoes the ingestion of gluten, a protein present in wheat, barley, rye, and products derived from these grains. This diet is necessary for both people with non-celiac gluten sensitivity and those with celiac disease, an autoimmune condition.

Consuming naturally gluten-free foods such as fruits, vegetables, legumes, nuts, seeds, dairy products, meat, and fish, as well as gluten-free grains (like rice, quinoa, corn, and millet), is a key component of gluten-free diets. These days, a variety of gluten-free options manufactured from different grains like buckwheat, amaranth, or sorghum are readily available for products like bread, pasta, and flour.

People who follow a gluten-free diet should carefully read food labels because gluten can hide in a variety of products, including processed foods, soups, sauces, and even some pharmaceuticals and cosmetics. Cross-contaminated foods, which occur when gluten-free products come into contact with gluten-containing ingredients during production or processing, may also contain gluten.

While a well-planned gluten-free diet can be nutritionally balanced, it's crucial to focus on some nutrients that may be missing as a result of cutting out gluten-containing grains. These nutrients include calcium, iron, zinc, B vitamins, fiber, and fiber. By including gluten-free whole grains, fortified gluten-free goods, a variety of fruits and vegetables, and protein sources, one can ensure an appropriate intake of these nutrients.

It is advised to speak with a healthcare provider or trained dietitian if you believe you may have celiac disease or gluten sensitivity. They can offer the right direction, support, and advice that are tailored to your particular requirements.

Dietary allergies

Food allergies are immune system reactions that happen as a result of the body mistaking some foods for being dangerous. From minor symptoms to severe, potentially fatal allergic reactions known as anaphylaxis, these reactions can vary widely. Peanuts, tree nuts, milk, eggs, soy, wheat, fish, and shellfish are among the common food allergies.

In order to prevent allergic responses, managing food allergies entails careful avoidance of the allergenic food(s). It's essential to carefully read food labels and be alert to any hazards of cross-contamination that can exist while food is being prepared. In rare circumstances, allergens can cause a reaction even in minute amounts.

It is crucial for people who have food allergies to get advice from a medical practitioner or certified dietician. They can assist in creating a healthy, balanced diet that is free of allergies and provides appropriate nourishment. To satisfy nutrient requirements, nutritional alternatives and different dietary selections can be suggested.

Food allergies can occasionally lead to dietary limitations or nutrient deficits. For instance, people who refuse milk may need alternate calcium sources, while people who avoid wheat may need adequate alternatives to grains that contain gluten. A dietician can offer advice on choosing healthy foods and, if necessary, suggest supplements.

Additionally, people who have a history of anaphylaxis or severe food allergies may need to carry emergency drugs (such as epinephrine auto-injectors) and learn how to administer them in case of unintentional allergen exposure.

A healthcare expert should be consulted if you believe you may have a food allergy in order to receive a proper diagnosis and management strategy.

Storing food properly

Maintaining food's quality, retaining its freshness, and limiting the development of dangerous germs that can lead to foodborne illnesses all depend on proper storage. Following are some broad suggestions for food storage:

1. **Refrigeration**: To ensure the safety and

freshness of perishable goods, store them in the refrigerator, including leftovers, raw meat, poultry, fish, dairy products, and other perishable items.
To stop bacteria from growing quickly, make sure the refrigerator is set at a temperature below 40°F (4°C).

To stop juices from spilling onto other foods, store raw meats and poultry in a drawer or on the lowest shelf possible.
Before refrigerating cooked items, place them in airtight containers.
In order to ensure optimum air circulation, don't overcrowd the refrigerator.
2. **Freezing**: Freezing has been shown to increase the shelf life of numerous goods. Foods should be packaged in freezer-safe containers or bags to prevent freezer burn and smells.
To track the freshness of items, make sure they are correctly labeled with the name

and date.

For optimal results, use the freezer right away. Food shouldn't be kept in the freezer for too long.

3. **Pantry and Dry Storage:** Keep canned goods, grains, cereals, pasta, and other dry items in a cold, dry, and dark pantry or closet.

Verify the use-by dates on items and move the older ones to the front for quicker use. To protect the products' quality and keep moisture and insects out, use airtight containers.

4. **Food Separation and Interference:** Prevent cross-contamination by keeping raw meat, poultry, and shellfish apart from meals that are ready to eat. Utilize distinct cutting boards and tools.

Keep raw meats in tight bags or containers to prevent drips or leaks that could contaminate other items.

To prevent odor transfer to other meals,

adequately wrap or seal goods with strong aromas, such as onions or garlic.

5. **Remains**: Immediately store leftovers in the fridge or freezer within two hours of cooking to stop bacterial growth. To help them cool quickly and evenly, store leftovers in shallow containers. Eat up any leftovers that are in the fridge within 3 to 4 days, or freeze them for later use.

Following precise storage instructions for various food items is crucial, as is being aware of any recommendations or guidelines supplied by food makers. You can reduce food waste, preserve food quality, and guarantee the safety of your family's food by storing it appropriately.

Preparation of food safely

Safe food preparation procedures are crucial for preventing foodborne infections and ensuring people's health and wellbeing.

Some crucial recommendations for preparing food safely are listed below:
Wash your hands thoroughly with soap and warm water for at least 20 seconds before handling food, after using the restroom, petting animals, or handling raw foods. Before and after usage, wash and sterilize kitchen counters, utensils, and cutting boards. For efficient cleaning, clean surfaces with hot, soapy water and a bleach solution.

Even if you want to peel the produce, wash fruits and vegetables under running water. To prevent cross-contamination, keep raw meat, poultry, seafood, and their juices away from meals that are ready to consume.

2. **Appropriate Food Preparation**: Cook meals sufficiently to eradicate dangerous microorganisms. For accurate measurement of interior temperatures, use a food

thermometer.

For chicken: 165°F (74°C).

Ground meats: 71°C (160°F)

For fish and other foods, 145°F (63°C)

145°F (63°C): Pork, veal, and lamb

145°F (63°C) (for medium-rare to medium) for steaks, roasts, and fish

3. Averting the Temperature Danger Zone: Keep perishable items away from the danger zone, which is between 40°F (4°C) and 140°F (60°C). In this region, bacteria proliferate quickly. Perishable meals should be stored quickly in the refrigerator or freezer, especially those that have been cooked or partially consumed.

4. **Safe Leftover Handling**: To minimize bacterial growth, store leftover food in the refrigerator or freezer within two hours of cooking.

To help them chill more quickly, divide

large portions of leftovers into smaller, shallow containers.

Before ingesting leftovers, reheat them to at least 165°F (74°C).

5. **Avoid eating raw or undercooked eggs**: Safe Handling of Raw Eggs and Dairy Cook eggs until the whites and yolks are set. To avoid spoilage, store perishable dairy items like milk, yogurt, and cheese in the refrigerator.

6. **Cleanliness Best Practices**: When preparing meals, stay away from touching your face, hair, or other surfaces. Separate chopping boards and utensils should be used for raw meat, poultry, shellfish, and prepared dishes. Use a tissue or your elbow to cover your mouth and nose when you cough or sneeze. Refrain from cooking food for others if you have gastrointestinal issues.

7. Adhere to the recommended temperature for food storage and expiration dates, and

observe the dates on food packaging. Use older food products before fresh ones to prevent spoiled food by adhering to the "first in, first out" concept.

The World Health Organization (WHO) and the Centers for Disease Control and Prevention (CDC) are two reputable sources that should be followed in addition to these recommendations if you want to prepare food safely. You can reduce your chance of contracting a foodborne illness and improve your own and others' health by using safe food preparation techniques.

Chapter 3

Prevention of Foodborne Diseases

For excellent health, foodborne infections must be avoided. Here are some crucial measures to avoid contracting a foodborne illness:

1. **Cleanliness**: Before handling food, thoroughly wash your hands with soap and warm water. This is especially important after visiting the restroom, handling pets, or touching raw foods. For at least 20 seconds, wash your hands.

Before and after usage, wash and sterilize kitchen counters, utensils, and cutting boards.

Even if you want to peel the produce, rinse it thoroughly under running water.

2. **Distancing**: To prevent cross-contamination, keep raw meat, poultry, seafood, and their juices away from meals

that are ready to consume.
For raw and cooked meals, use different cutting boards, cutlery, and plates.
To prevent their juices from contaminating other items, store raw meats in sealed containers or bags.
3. **Appropriate Cooking**: Cook meals sufficiently to eradicate dangerous microorganisms. Make sure internal temperatures are met by using a food thermometer.
For chicken: 165°F (74°C).
Ground meats: 71°C (160°F)
For fish and other foods, 145°F (63°C)
145°F (63°C): Pork, veal, and lamb
145°F (63°C) (for medium-rare to medium) for steaks, roasts, and fish
4. **Maintain proper temperature**: Keep perishable items out of the danger zone (40°F to 140°F or 4°C to 60°C), where bacteria can quickly proliferate.
Quickly refrigerate perishable foods, and

make sure your refrigerator is set to 40°F (4°C) or lower.

Use the microwave, a refrigerator, or cold running water to thaw frozen items. At room temperature, do not defrost.

5. **Safe Leftover Handling**: Within two hours of cooking, store leftovers in the refrigerator or freezer.

To cool leftovers more quickly in the fridge, divide big servings into smaller, shallow containers.

Before ingesting leftovers, reheat them to at least 165°F (74°C).

6. **Trustworthy Sources**: Shop at respected stores and marketplaces, and make sure that the food is handled and stored properly. Make sure that canned foods are in good shape and refrain from utilizing cans that have leaks, bulges, or dents.

7. **Foods to Avoid**: Avoid foods that pose a risk, such as raw or undercooked eggs, raw sprouts, unpasteurized dairy products, and

raw or undercooked shellfish. Refrain from eating food that has raw or undercooked ingredients, such as homemade Caesar dressing or cookie dough.

8. **Remain Informed**: Stay informed about food recalls and safety alerts issued by regulatory or health entities. comply with expiration dates and recommended storage methods for food.

You can dramatically lower your chance of contracting a foodborne illness by adhering to these recommendations. It's crucial to keep your kitchen clean and use the right cooking methods. It's also important to be aware of food safety procedures.

A heart-healthy diet

An essential part of preserving cardiovascular health and lowering the risk of heart disease is eating a heart-healthy diet. A heart-healthy diet can be summarized as follows:

1. **Place a priority on fruits and vegetables**: Try to include a range of fruits and vegetables in your meals. These supply important antioxidants, vitamins, and minerals.

Juices frequently contain additional sugars and have less fiber than whole fruits and vegetables, so choose the latter instead. Leafy greens, berries, citrus fruits, and cruciferous vegetables are some examples of colorful food choices.

Place a priority on whole grains by substituting them for processed grains in your diet. Fiber-rich whole grains can reduce cholesterol levels because of their high fiber content. Consider full-grain bread and pasta, brown rice, oats, quinoa, and whole wheat as possibilities.

Include lean proteins in your diet to reduce your intake of saturated fats. Legumes, nuts, seeds, skinless poultry, fish (particularly oily fish like salmon or mackerel high in omega-3 fatty acids), and fish are all healthy options.

Limit your intake of processed foods, red meat, and dairy items with added fat.

4. **Healthy Fats**: Choose heart-healthy fats when possible. Monounsaturated fats, such as those in olive oil, avocados, and nuts, as well as polyunsaturated fats, like those in flaxseeds, walnuts, and fatty fish, are among these.

Reduce the consumption of fried foods, processed snacks, and animal products that are high in saturated and trans fats.

5. Reduce your sodium consumption to help keep your blood pressure in a healthy range. Eat less salt and choose low-sodium options by avoiding adding excess salt to your meals.

Observe the salt content in packaged and processed foods. Wherever possible, choose fresh or home-cooked meals.

6. Limit your intake of processed foods, sweetened beverages, and sweets that include added sugars. Limit the use of processed sugars in baking and cooking and choose natural sweeteners like fruits.

7. Moderate Alcohol Consumption: If you drink, do it in moderation. Typically speaking, this entails a maximum of one drink for ladies and two for men per day. Noting that abstainers shouldn't start drinking for prospective health advantages is crucial.

8. **Maintain Quantity amounts**: To keep your weight in check, pay attention to your portion amounts. Consider using smaller bowls and plates, and be careful of high-calorie foods.

9. **Maintain Hydration:** To maintain hydration and promote general health, drink lots of water throughout the day.

It's important to keep in mind that every person's dietary requirements are unique, so it's advised to speak with a healthcare provider or certified dietitian to create a heart-healthy diet plan that is tailored to your unique situation and medical needs.

Obesity and weight loss

A crucial component of overall health and wellbeing is managing weight and fighting obesity. An overview of methods for addressing obesity through diet and nutrition is given below:

1. **Caloric Balance**: To keep your weight in check, strike a balance between the calories you consume and the energy you expend. Consume the recommended number of calories for your age, sex, activity level, and goals.

To lose weight, if necessary, create a calorie deficit by combining a healthy diet with exercise.

Focus on a balanced diet that consists of a variety of nutrient-dense foods.

2. A balanced and Nutrient-Dense diet Incorporate fresh produce, nutritious grains, lean meats, and dairy items that are low in fat or fat-free.

Consume fewer processed, high-calorie, and nutritionally deficient items, such as sugary fast food, snacks, and beverages.

3. **Portion Control**: To prevent ingesting too many calories, be aware of portion proportions.

Make use of smaller plates and bowls, and be aware of your hunger and fullness cues.

Develop an understanding of proper serving sizes by practicing portion management by first measuring or weighing foods.

4. Mindful Consumption: Take your time while eating and focus on the flavors and textures of the meal.

Recognize when you are hungry and when you are full to prevent overeating.

Refrain from using electronic gadgets or watching television while you're eating.

5. **Establish Frequent Food Routines**: Avoid skipping meals and create regular meal routines.

Mix macronutrients, including proteins, healthy fats, and carbohydrates, throughout each meal.

Schedule meals in advance to lower the possibility that you'll make poor eating decisions out of boredom or lack of time.

6. **Physical Activity**: Exercise frequently to help you manage your weight and maintain good   health.

Include strength training activities together

with at least 150 minutes per week of moderate-to-strength aerobic activity.

7. **Behavior and Emotional Support**:
Seek assistance from medical specialists, licensed dietitians, or support groups that concentrate on weight management.
Address emotional eating and create coping mechanisms for handling stressful situations or emotional triggers.
To treat underlying psychological issues related to weight control, think about cognitive-behavioral therapy or behavioral counseling.

8. **Stable Lifestyle Improvements**: Rather than implementing tight diets or fast cures, put more of an emphasis on changing eating behaviors in a sustainable way. Make healthy eating habits and regular exercise a part of your lifestyle if you want to achieve long-term success. Track your progress while setting

reasonable targets and acknowledging even the smallest victories.

In order to create a personalized weight control strategy based on your unique requirements and medical conditions, it's crucial to speak with a healthcare expert or registered dietitian. In order to help you control your weight, they can offer individualized counseling and assistance.

Controlling one's weight and dealing with obesity

The prevention and treatment of obesity, as well as maintaining a healthy weight, are crucial to one's physical and mental health. The following is an overview of many ways to address obesity and manage one's weight in relation to diet and nutrition:

1. Maintaining a healthy weight requires striking a balance between the amount of calories consumed and the amount of energy

expended each day. Consume the right amount of calories for your age, gender, degree of activity, and weight loss objectives, taking all of these factors into account. If you need to lose weight, you should engage in a combination of a good diet and physical activity in order to generate a calorie deficit.

2. **Eat a Diet That Is Well-Balanced and Rich in Nutrients**: Make sure you eat a diet that is well-balanced and rich in nutrients, including a wide variety of foods. Include fruits, vegetables, lean proteins, whole grains, and dairy products that are low in fat or fat-free in your diet. Restrict your consumption of processed foods, high-calorie foods, and items that are high in calories but low in nutritional content, such as sugary snacks, fast food, and sugary beverages.

3. **Pay Attention to Portion Sizes**: If you want to avoid consuming an excessive amount of calories, pay attention to the sizes of the portions you are served. Make use of dishes and bowls that are smaller in size, and pay attention to your body's signs for when you are hungry and when you are full.

In the beginning, it is helpful to establish an awareness of acceptable serving sizes by practicing portion management by measuring or weighing food.

4. In order to practice mindful eating, one should eat slowly and pay attention to the sensations elicited by the food being consumed.

To keep from overeating, it is important to pay attention to the signals that your body sends you regarding hunger and fullness. It is best to eat without any distractions, such as the television or electronic devices, when you can.

5. Establish Regular Meal Patterns: It is important to establish regular meal patterns to prevent skipping meals. Make sure that every meal contains a balance of different types of macronutrients, such as carbohydrates, proteins, and healthy fats.

Having a meal plan will help you avoid making rash decisions about what to eat when you're hungry or pressed for time.

6. Participate in Regular Physical Activity: Taking part in regular physical activity is a great way to support healthy weight control and general health.

Aim to do at least 150 minutes of aerobic activity per week at a moderate intensity or 75 minutes of activity per week at a strong intensity, in addition to strength training exercises.

7. Support for Behavior and Emotional Well-Being: Seek support from healthcare professionals, licensed dietitians, or support groups that specialize in weight management.

Deal with emotional eating and work on developing coping mechanisms for dealing with stress or other emotional triggers. It may be beneficial to seek out behavioral counseling or cognitive-behavioral therapy in order to address the psychological reasons that are at the root of weight management.

8. Make Changes That Are Sustainable In Your Lifestyle: Instead of adopting restrictive diets or fast cures, put your attention on creating changes that are sustainable to your eating habits.

Your goal should be to be successful over the long run by adopting good eating patterns and regular physical activity into your lifestyle.

Specify attainable objectives, keep tabs on

your development, and reward yourself for reaching even the smallest milestones along the road.

It is crucial to build a tailored plan for weight management based on your specific needs and health concerns by consulting with a healthcare expert or a certified dietitian as part of this process. They are able to offer you individualized advice and assistance throughout your quest to manage your weight.

Chapter 4

Nutritional needs during pregnancy
It is extremely important for both the mother's health and the baby's development for her to have the appropriate nourishment throughout her pregnancy. The following is a list of important things to think about and rules to follow in order to keep a healthy diet while expecting:

1. **Consume a Diet That Is Well-Balanced**: Consume a diet that is well-balanced and consists of a variety of foods that are rich in nutrients to ensure that you achieve your nutritional requirements. Include in your meals a variety of fruits, vegetables, whole grains, lean proteins, dairy products or alternatives to dairy products, and healthy fats.
2. **Folate and Folic Acid**: An adequate consumption of folate and folic acid in the

first few weeks of pregnancy is essential for assisting in the prevention of neural tube abnormalities.

Include folic acid-rich foods in your diet, including citrus fruits, legumes, leafy greens, and cereals that have been fortified with folic acid. Folic acid is also found in some prenatal vitamins.

3. **Iron**: Iron is an essential component in the formation of red blood cells and helps protect pregnant women from developing anemia.

Include in your diet foods that are high in the mineral iron, such as lean meats, poultry, fish, legumes, cereals with added iron, and dark green leafy vegetables. Consuming foods that are high in vitamin C, such as citrus fruits, can help improve the body's ability to absorb iron.

4. **Calcium and Vitamin D:** Adequate consumption of calcium and vitamin D is essential for the development of the

mother's fetus' bones and also contributes to the preservation of the mother's bone health. You should incorporate salmon, tofu, leafy greens, dairy products, and plant-based milks that have been fortified into your diet. Additionally, time spent outdoors in the sun is necessary for the production of vitamin D. If you don't get much sun, you might want to consider taking a vitamin D supplement.

5. **Omega-3 Fatty Acids**: Omega-3 fatty acids, in particular docosahexaenoic acid (also known as DHA), are essential for the development of the brain and eyes in developing fetuses.
Include in your diet sources of omega-3 fatty acids such as fatty fish (for example, salmon and sardines), chia seeds, flaxseeds, and walnuts. Some prenatal vitamins also provide DHA.

6. **Protein**: Consuming an adequate amount of protein helps promote the growth and

development of tissues in both the mother and the infant when enough amounts are consumed.

Incorporate into your diet lean cuts of meat, poultry, fish, eggs, legumes, nuts, and seeds, as well as dairy products or alternatives to dairy products.

7. **Hydration**: In order to keep your body well hydrated and to ensure that it can carry out its tasks, you should drink a lot of water throughout the day.

8. **Adopt Safe Food Handling**: In order to prevent foodborne infections that can be harmful to both the mother and the infant, it is important to practice safe food handling. This includes the correct storage, preparation, and cooking of food. Steer clear of eating meats, fish, or eggs that are uncooked or undercooked. Additionally, use extreme caution when consuming unpasteurized dairy products as well as certain kinds of seafood.

9. **Personalized Directions**: Speak with a medical expert or a registered dietitian who is an expert in pregnancy nutrition. Speak with someone who is knowledgeable about breastfeeding. They are able to provide individualized suggestions that are based on your specific needs, which may include dietary restrictions or worries about your health.

It is essential to keep in mind that there is no "typical" pregnancy and that each woman's nutritional requirements may be different. During pregnancy, maintaining open contact with one's healthcare providers and going to prenatal checkups on a consistent basis are two of the best ways to guarantee that both the mother and the baby are in the best possible health.

Provision of nourishment for newborns and children of preschool age

It is essential for an infant's and young

child's growth, development, and overall health to receive the appropriate nutrition during the infant and toddler years. The following are some important things to keep in mind and suggestions with regard to the diet of newborns and young children:

1. **Breastfeeding and/or Formula Feeding**: Breast milk is the best source of nutrition for infants. Formula can be used in addition to breastfeeding. It supplies all of the essential nutrients and antibodies and also encourages the formation of bonds. If you are unable to breastfeed your child, an alternate option is using infant formula that is specifically formulated for their age. Be sure to adhere to the necessary dietary guidelines that are prescribed by medical professionals.

2. **Start Introducing Basic foods:**
Gradually Start introducing solid foods at the age of 6 months while continuing to breastfeed or use formula.

Start with foods that are high in iron, such as baby cereals that have been enriched with iron, pureed meats, chicken, or lentils. Introduce the newborn to a wide range of fruits, vegetables, whole grains, and other sources of protein in stages, taking into account the infant's capacity for handling new foods and their readiness to develop.

3. Encourage Self-Feeding and the investigation of Age-Appropriate Finger foods. As newborns develop, it is important to encourage self-feeding and the investigation of age-appropriate finger foods.

Provide items that are tender and simple to manipulate, such as prepared vegetables and fruits, little bits of tender meat, or tofu.

4. Provide a range of Nutrient-Dense meals: In order to meet the developing child's nutritional needs, it is important to provide a range of meals that are high in nutrients. Include in their meals a variety of fruits,

vegetables, lean proteins (such as chicken, fish, eggs, and lentils), whole grains, dairy products or alternatives to dairy products, and healthy fats.

5. **Allergic Foods**: When introducing potentially allergic foods, do so in a slow and methodical manner, one at a time, while following the advice of healthcare specialists.

Peanuts, tree nuts, eggs, milk, fish, shellfish, wheat, and soy are examples of foods that frequently cause allergic reactions in people.

It is essential to keep an eye out for any allergic reactions and seek professional medical assistance.

6. **Stay Away from Added Sugar and Salt**: In the diets of newborns and young children, it is important to minimize or eliminate the amount of added sugar and salt. It is best not to provide sweet beverages and foods that are heavy in added sugars.

Reduce the amount of salt and salty seasonings you use in cooking, and stay away from highly processed meals that are high in sodium.

7. **Hydration**: As the child gets older, you should start giving him or her water in addition to breast milk or formula. Avoid offering fruit juices and other beverages with added sugar to newborns who have not yet reached their first birthday.

8. **Establishing a Favorable Eating Environment and Serving as a Role Model**: In order to establish a favorable eating environment, have frequent meals with your family and maintain a laid-back setting.

Be a good example for others by demonstrating healthy eating behaviors such as eating a variety of foods and taking pleasure in eating fruits and vegetables.

9. **Scheduling Routine Examinations and Consultations:** Maintain routine checkups with your healthcare providers in order to have your development monitored, be evaluated, and receive nutritional advice. Consult with the child's physician or a qualified dietitian in order to receive individualized recommendations tailored to the child's requirements as well as any particular dietary issues.

Because of this, the nutritional requirements of each child may be different. It is essential to seek the advice of trained medical professionals in order to guarantee that newborns and young children receive the necessary nutrition and to support healthy growth and development.

The importance of nutrition for adult
It is absolutely necessary for older folks to consume the appropriate nutrients in order

to keep their health and well-being in good standing. The following is a list of some of the most important things to keep in mind and some advice regarding diet for this population:

1. **Consume a Diet That Is Well-Balanced:** It is important to eat a diet that is well-balanced and that consists of a wide variety of foods that are rich in nutrients. Place an emphasis on eating fruits, vegetables, whole grains, lean proteins (such as chicken, fish, and lentils), dairy products or substitutes that are low in fat or fat-free, and healthy fats.

2. **Consumption of an Adequate Amount of Fiber:** Make certain that you consume an adequate amount of fiber by consuming whole grains, fruits, vegetables, legumes, and nuts.

The consumption of fiber is beneficial to one's digestive health, as it assists in the regulation of bowel movements and enhances one's cardiovascular health.

3. **Consume an Adequate Amount of Protein**: Ensure that your diet has an adequate amount of protein by consuming foods like lean meats, poultry, fish, eggs, dairy products or substitutes, legumes, and nuts.

It is absolutely necessary to consume a sufficient amount of protein in order to maintain one's muscular mass, strength, and overall health.

4. **Calcium and Vitamin D**: In order to maintain healthy bones, it is important to get an adequate amount of calcium and vitamin D from your diet.

Include in your diet foods such as plant-based milk that has been fortified, dairy products, leafy green vegetables, and fish with bones that can be eaten.

If necessary, vitamin D can also be

supplied through the use of dietary supplements in addition to sun exposure.

5. **Hydration:** In order to keep your body properly hydrated throughout the day, you should make sure to drink a suitable amount of water as well as other fluids. The danger of dehydration may be greater in elderly people; therefore, maintaining proper hydration is essential for the proper functioning of many organs and systems in the body.

6. **Adequate Vitamin B12**: Ensure that you are getting an adequate amount of vitamin B12 in your diet. This may be more difficult for older people to do because of their diminished ability to absorb the vitamin.

Ensure that your diet consists of a variety of foods, such as cereals that have been fortified, as well as meat, fish, poultry, and dairy products.

Supplements may be required, particularly

for individuals who have deficits that have been clinically determined.

7. **Decrease Your Sodium Intake**: In order to improve the health of your cardiovascular system, you should lower the amount of sodium that you consume. Reduce the amount of processed meals, canned products, and fast food that you eat because these types of foods typically contain high amounts of salt. Instead of salting food, try seasoning it with herbs and spices, and whenever possible, go for low-sodium substitutes.

8. **Participate in Regular Physical Activity**: It is important to participate in regular physical activity as it is recommended by medical authorities. Participating in physical activity is beneficial to one's general health as well as their mobility, muscle strength, and bone health.

9. **Enhancing Your Physical, Emotional, and Social Well-Being**: Enhancing your physical, emotional, and social well-being by maintaining social relationships around food and sharing meals with others can help boost your enjoyment of food and your appetite.

Deal with any issues relating to your mental or emotional health that may be causing you to lose control of your eating habits and your nutritional well-being.

10. **Scheduling Frequent Appointments for Checkups and Consultations:** It is highly recommended that checkups, screenings, and nutritional assessments be conducted at regular intervals by qualified medical specialists.

Consult with certified dietitians or healthcare experts for individualized suggestions that are based on individual needs, health circumstances, and any particular dietary concerns.

It is vitally important for older people to construct tailored nutrition regimens in consultation with healthcare providers or registered dietitians. They are able to provide specialist advice and assistance in tackling any one-of-a-kind issues or particular health conditions.

Chapter 5

Eating well on a limited spending plan Consuming a healthy diet while adhering to a financial constraint can be difficult, but it is unquestionably doable with a little bit of forethought and some astute decisions. Here are some suggestions for eating healthily while remaining frugal:

1. **Make a food plan**: Developing a meal plan for the week is an excellent way to both save money and guarantee that you are eating meals that are high in nutrition. To get started, compile a list of dishes that you enjoy that are straightforward and easy on the wallet, and then make a grocery list based on the items required.

2. **Purchase in large quantities**: One way to save money on food expenses is to buy staple foods in large quantities, such as grains, pasta, beans, and frozen fruits and

vegetables. These ingredients have a longer shelf life and are versatile enough to be utilized in a variety of different dishes.

3. **Prepare meals at home**: Eating out or getting takeout can quickly add up to a significant amount of money. When you cook at home, you can control the portion sizes, use healthier foods, and save money all at the same time. Try your hand at recreating some of your favorite dishes from local restaurants at home.

4. **Shop for food that is in season**: You should choose to buy fruits and vegetables that are in season because they are typically less expensive and more easily available when they are at their peak harvest times. The best bargains can be found at farmer's markets and other local product booths.

5. Make use of any leftovers by repurposing them into new dishes using your imagination and leftovers. For instance, you can add leftover roasted chicken to salads or

sandwiches, and you can combine overripe fruits into smoothies or use them in baking. There are countless ways to repurpose food.

6. Decrease your consumption of meat; given the high cost of meat, you might consider increasing your consumption of proteins derived from plants. Alternatives that are both inexpensive and versatile, such as beans, lentils, tofu, and eggs, can be utilized to make a wide variety of recipes.

7. Compare prices at multiple local stores in order to obtain the best offers before making a purchase of food by doing a price comparison at several different local retailers. Think about using coupons or downloading apps that provide savings opportunities.

8. Restrict your consumption of processed foods. Snacks and other convenience foods that have been processed are typically more

expensive and offer little in the way of nutritional value. Instead, go for entire meals like fruits, vegetables, nuts, and grains that are still in their original form.

9. Make your meals in advance, as cooking in bulk and planning meals in advance will help you save both time and money. Prepare meals in large quantities and store them in an appropriate manner for subsequent usage. This way, you won't be tempted to eat out as often because you'll always have nutritious options within easy reach in your home.

10. Drink plenty of water to stay hydrated instead of sugary beverages such as soda and juice, which may be both expensive and unhealthy. Stick to water as your beverage of choice because it is not only the least expensive option but also the one that will hydrate you the most effectively. Keep in mind that maintaining a healthy diet

does not have to be prohibitively expensive. You are able to stick to a budget while still consuming a nutritious diet if you plan ahead, do your shopping strategically, and make mindful food selections.

Planning and preparing meals as it relates to food and nutrition

The maintenance of a healthy diet requires meticulous attention to both the planning and preparation of one's meals. The following are some suggestions that will assist you in the planning and preparation of your meals:

1. Set aside time for planning: Each week, designate a particular day or time for the purpose of organizing your meals. When developing your meal plan, it is important to take into account not only your schedule but also your dietary requirements and preferences.

2. Create a menu for the week that includes breakfast, lunch, dinner, and snacks. Start by creating a menu for the week that includes breakfast, lunch, and dinner. Be careful to incorporate a wide variety of fruits, vegetables, whole grains, lean meats, and healthy fats into your diet in order to achieve a good balance of nutrients.

3. **Compile a shopping list**: Using the menu as a guide, compile a comprehensive shopping list of all the items you'll need to complete the meal. Check your refrigerator and pantry to see what food and drink you already have so that you can avoid buying the same thing twice.

4. **Make smart purchases:** When you go shopping, bring a grocery list with you and stick to it. This will help you avoid making impulsive purchases. Make sure to eat plenty of fresh produce, lean meats,

nutritious grains, and dairy items that are low in fat. If you want to find the best bargains, you might think about shopping at local markets or using online food delivery services.

5. Prepare what you need ahead of time. In order to save time during the week, you should begin preparing the components as soon as you bring the groceries into the house. Prepare foods such as grains and legumes to be stored in the refrigerator for later use by chopping vegetables, marinating meats, and cooking grains.

6. Prepare larger quantities of certain dishes, such as soups, stews, or casseroles, that can then be portioned out into individual servings and frozen. This technique is referred to as batch cooking. On hectic days, you'll be able to grab and go with these meals that are already prepared.

7. Pay attention to the size of your portions while you prepare your food so that you can guarantee that you are getting the appropriate number of calories each day. To accurately portion out the right amounts, you can make use of measuring cups, food scales, or visual cues.

8. **Correctly store food**: When it comes to correctly storing your prepared goods and meals, you should consider making an investment in freezer-safe bags or airtight containers. You should write the date on the label to ensure that you use them within the appropriate window of time.

9. Create adaptable components that may be used in a variety of ways throughout the week by mixing and matching them. For instance, you may prepare a large quantity of quinoa that can be used as a side dish, in salads, or even in stir-fries.

10. Maintain organization by writing down your food plan and storing recipes in a notebook or using an app that does meal planning. This will help you keep organized and prevent you from making any hasty judgments that might not be in line with the health goals you have set for yourself.

Time may be saved, stress can be reduced, and a healthy diet can be maintained if you follow these suggestions for the planning and preparation of meals. You can maintain the excitement and enjoyment of your meals by experimenting with a variety of flavors and dishes.

Eating healthfully in terms of diet and nutrition

When you're trying to stick to a healthy diet, maintaining a healthy diet while dining out might be difficult, but there are strategies to make better choices. Here are some helpful hints for making good decisions when dining out:

1. Do some research on the menu ahead of time: Before going to the restaurant, look the menu up on the internet. This enables you to plan ahead and select options that are better for your health. Keep an eye out for meals that incorporate lean proteins, nutritious grains, and a generous helping of vegetables.

2. Pick the correct restaurant: When looking for a new place to eat, prioritize establishments that feature fresh, whole foods or offer a variety of healthy menu options. Choices that are healthier, lower in calories, vegetarian, or vegan are becoming increasingly common at restaurants.

3. Watch the size of your dishes: Restaurants typically serve larger amounts, which might lead to consuming too much

food. Think about ordering a dish with a buddy and sharing it, or ask for a takeout container when your food comes out. Remove a suitable quantity and save the remaining food aside for a later time.

4. Pay attention to the techniques of preparation: go for foods that are baked, grilled, steamed, or roasted rather than those that are fried or sautéed. In general, these cooking methods require less oil and are better for you as a result.

5. Alter your order. Don't be hesitant to ask for your order to be altered so that it meets your specific dietary requirements. Ask for the dressings and sauces to be served on the side; select lean proteins; go for the whole grain alternatives; and make sure to get extra vegetables.

6. Keep an eye on the additional sugars and fats: When it comes to dressings, sauces, and condiments, watch out for those that

pack on extra calories that you don't need. Use them in moderation or ask for alternatives that are less heavy.

7. Pay attention to the beverages you consume. Calories can quickly build up when you drink sugary beverages such as soda, sweetened tea, or alcoholic beverages. If you want to make a healthier choice, go for water, unsweetened tea, or sparkling water with a slice of lemon.

8. Give priority to veggies: If you want to fill up on vegetables, request a side salad or ask for extra vegetables to be included in your main dish. They supply necessary nutrients and have the ability to make you feel fuller without causing you to overeat.

9. Chew your food more slowly and relish each bite. When you practice mindful eating, you slow down your eating pace, taste each meal, and pay attention to your

body's signs for when it is hungry and when it is full. This can assist in preventing you from overeating and allow you to take fuller pleasure in the food that you eat.

10. If you are attempting to eat healthier, do not order the breadbasket, appetizers, or dessert. These add-ons frequently provide surplus calories and make it more difficult to maintain your desired nutritional intake. Always keep in mind that going out to eat does not mean you have to abandon your efforts to maintain a balanced diet. You are able to savor a meal at a restaurant while still staying on track to achieve your objectives if you choose foods carefully, pay attention to the sizes of your portions, and give the most weight to the nutrient-dense options.

Summary

Food and nutrition are key components of our lives that have a significant impact on our health and well-being in a variety of different ways. It is essential to both one's physical and mental health to consume a diet that is well-rounded and contains a wide variety of foods that are rich in nutrients. While macronutrients (proteins, carbs, and fats) are the primary sources of energy, micronutrients (vitamins and minerals) play an important role in maintaining a wide variety of body processes. When we eat a wide variety of fruits, vegetables, whole grains, lean proteins, and healthy fats, we obtain the important vitamins, minerals, antioxidants, and fiber that we need, which is good for our cardiovascular system, brain, digestion, and metabolic processes.

Keeping a healthy weight and getting the most out of one's diet also requires practicing portion management, meal planning, and various cooking techniques.

A healthier relationship with food can be fostered through the practice of mindful eating as well as an understanding of food labels. In addition, for the health of the earth, it is necessary to take into consideration issues of sustainability, food source, and food safety. If you put an emphasis on food and nutrition, you will notice an increase in energy, an improvement in your immunity, an improvement in your mood, and an overall improvement in your well-being.

Conclusion

In conclusion, food and nutrition are of the utmost significance in our lives since they have an impact on our health, vitality, and overall quality of life. It is essential to eat a diet that is both well-balanced and contains a wide variety of foods that are rich in nutrients in order to supply our bodies with the fuel and building blocks they require for optimal operation. It is possible for us to ensure that we acquire the necessary vitamins, minerals, antioxidants, and fiber for a healthy body and mind if we consume a wide variety of fruits, vegetables, whole grains, lean meats, and healthy fats.

Food and nutrition have a far-reaching influence on different elements of our well-being, beyond just their role as a source of sustenance. A diet that is adequate provides support for our immune system, guards against chronic diseases, enhances brain function, improves heart health, facilitates digestion, speeds up metabolism, and helps contribute to improved energy levels. It also plays a key role in the control and maintenance of one's weight.

The cultivation of good eating habits, such as portion management, meal planning, and mindful eating, equips us with the ability to make educated decisions regarding our nutrition and assists us in preserving a healthy connection with food. In addition, knowing where our food comes from, taking into account issues of sustainability, and ensuring that it is safe to eat gives us the power to make decisions that are both morally and environmentally responsible regarding the food that we consume.

We will be able to realize the promise of greater overall well-being and a higher quality of life if we make food and nutrition a priority.he practice of providing our bodies with the appropriate nutrition is not only beneficial to us physiologically, but it also supports our mental and emotional well-being. We may achieve optimal health, longevity, and a harmonious relationship with both our bodies and the world that surrounds us if we combine the principles of adequate nutrition, mindful eating practices, and a sustainable approach to food.

www.ingramcontent.com/pod-product-compliance
Lightning Source LLC
Chambersburg PA
CBHW050044260726
48658CB00005B/1767